Mental Health: My story of Coping

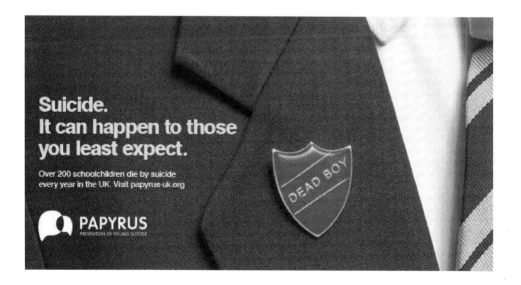

Suicide.
It can happen to those
you least expect.

Over 200 schoolchildren die by suicide
every year in the UK. Visit papyrus-uk.org

PAPYRUS
PREVENTION OF YOUNG SUICIDE

CONTENTS:

INTRODUCTION: LIVING WITH DOMESTIC ABUSE

My first experience of violence was from my dad beating me, my siblings and my mum mercilessly. The whole family was afraid of him and what he would do if we did anything that he considered was wrong. This resulted from the fact that my father was an abusive alcoholic. Every day he would drink alcohol until he was unconscious. This was one of the only times during the day we felt safe. When he regained consciousness, he would drink again until he became unconscious once more.

He used to find things to physically abuse us with. These would include belts and slippers, or shoes and my mum would have to pull him off us because he would not stop. This abuse had been continuous for the first 9 years of my life. Admittedly, I had it slightly easier than my siblings because I was my father's favorite child. He always called my sister a mistake and would always find fault in anything she did.

We lived in a country in the Middle East called Oman. It was forbidden by his religion to consume alcohol. This, however, made no difference to him. He had cheated on my mum on multiple occasions with the housemaids and with hired prostitutes. He would knowingly drink-drive with the whole family in the car on a regular basis and we dared not contradict him. My father also used to verbally abuse the housemaids if the job they had done didn't meet his standards.

My siblings and I never brought friends home because he wouldn't allow it. Due to this, I grew up with mostly the house maids as my friends. When they left to go back to their own country, whether it was to visit their family permanently, I would always cry because I had no control over losing my only friends. At the time this life felt normal because it was all I ever knew.

My father was basically an intelligent man but was ruined by his addiction to alcohol. He had been taken to rehabilitation centers on 3 separate occasions but couldn't get rid of the addiction. He was a hydrocarbon accountant and mechanical engineer for Shell based at the Petroleum Development of Oman but eventually lost his job because he was always drunk. The addiction had completely consumed his life. I have never seen him sober.

However, there was no escape from the violence because when we were taken to school, teachers would hit us and throw things at us. The reasoning for this would be as simple as incorrectly answering a question. Every incident was denied when confronted by my mum regardless of the marks and bruises we were left with due to the issue.

My father had arrived to visit us in a blue 2008 VW Golf which, he had hired from Sixt. We had seen that there was damage on the bonnet of the vehicle and all the way along the roof. He insisted that he had collided with a traffic cone. However, we are all, to this day, convinced he had a road traffic collision with a pedestrian due to being too inebriated to adequately focus on the road whilst driving. When returning to Oman, he did not return the vehicle to Sixt. Instead, he had abandoned the vehicle in the multi-story parking lot at terminal 3 of Heathrow Airport.

All the abuse and the addiction to alcohol had caused my mum to move back to England and divorce my father. My father stayed in Oman. However, things seemed to take a turn for the worst when this happened.

CHAPTER 1: THE DIVORCE

Initially, living in England we were made to move into an apartment above an estate agent in a small seaside town in Essex. This apartment was filled with mould and rising damp and regularly made us ill due to the poor living conditions but during this period, we had no alternative option. For a few weeks, we had no furniture apart from a cushion on the floor in the reception room of this apartment. Overnight, we would sleep on the floor and sometimes have to go to a relative's house for dinner because we had no means of making any food.

At this time, my father was unaware that my mum had planned to divorce him, and he bought her a car and some furniture for the apartment. My brother and I didn't know that she had planned to leave him at this point either. One day, he had arrived at my school to pick me up and as we got back to the apartment, he fell through the window of the estate agents' office below and cut his head and arm because he was drunk. He was made to pay for the damage and then returned to Oman to continue working.

When my mum began taking the necessary legal action to proceed to a divorce, my father had then returned to England in an attempt to take my brother and me back with him. My mum had refused to let this happen for our safety, and at some point, extreme measures had to be taken in order to counteract the extreme inhumane acts he was carrying out in order to achieve his goal.

At the time that we became aware of his arrival in England we had to depart the apartment with some of our belongings and stay in a hotel. He didn't know that we had gone to stay in a hotel for a while but, had decided to break the glass next to the door to gain entry to the apartment. Once he had gained entry and saw that there were clothes everywhere and one of the suitcases were gone, he came to the realisation that we had vacated the apartment for a while in order to avoid the danger to our lives that we were all facing.

He had called my mum and made threats to kill her in order to abduct us and to commit suicide had she carried through with the divorce and not given us over to him. This information was handed to the police who had assigned us a constable with the Domestic Violence Unit of Essex Police. Feeling a little more at ease, we had been returned to school. With the instructions provided to the schools to call the police if my father was on their premises and not to allow him to pick us up. He was then to be arrested for attempted abduction if this situation arises.

On my first day back at school, I was escorted to reception to 2 waiting police officers around 1 hour early because my father had been seen on site. My mum was called to pick me up but had sent my grandmother because she couldn't come. He was arrested and later released on bail. As my grandmother and I returned to their ground floor apartment, I noticed my mum was crying and I instantly hugged my mum and asked what was wrong. She had taken me around the corner to where her car was parked. All the tyres had been cut and the windows were all smashed with dents all along the sides and front and back of the car. It had become apparent that someone had attacked the vehicle with a hammer. This was known because of the pattern of the break in the sun roof. It was evident that the hammer was broken through the glass, twisted and retracted again.

My mother had additionally, discovered that my father had cut up all her underwear and discarded it. He then made the statement "no other man will see my wife in her underwear".

The car had to be driven to the local repair garage because my mum could not afford to hire a tow truck to collect the car. My mum had insisted on visiting the apartment accompanied by the police and my aunt. Upon arrival, he was discovered sat on the armchair with an axe, a bottle of whiskey and a baseball bat waiting for her to arrive at the apartment. Once again, he was arrested and released on bail and the items were seized as evidence and later destroyed by Essex Police. My mum had to borrow my aunt's car because her car was still in for repairs from the extensive amount of damage which was caused to the vehicle. The repairs included but were not limited to, new glass for all windows, 4 new tyres and some body work and interior work for the car.

We returned to the hotel in the borrowed car. Due to the car being expensive to repair, we had only a small amount of money left. When we went for a breakfast buffet the next morning, my mum and sister took 2 empty bags and had to fill them up to make sure we could eat for the rest of the day. We had then needed to return to the apartment to get some clean clothes. Upon arrival at the apartment, a noose had been discovered hung above the stairs to the second level of the apartment which, had been left by my father. We were told by my mum not to touch it, who took pictures of it and called the police.

We then returned to the hotel. Upon arrival at school the next day, I had been told by my friends and my mum was told by the teachers that my father was seen on site and attempted to pick me up being unaware that I had not attended the school that day. They also said that there was a containment set up by the police surrounding the school and PSU (riot) van had parked inside the school premises whilst the officers were sent to search for him in the school premises. He was arrested once again and released on bail. He had decided to skip bail and leave the country to return to Oman. He was now wanted by Essex Police for skipping bail.

We had decided to move out urgently. We had moved into a house on the next street. When he returned to England, he bought a 3 door 1996 white Vauxhall Corsa which, he parked outside my grandmother's house in order to follow her and my grandfather to our new address. They passed this information on to my mum who had conveyed it straight to the police. He was arrested and charged for the offences of breaking and entering on multiple occasions, skipping bail, making threats to kill, criminal damage, being in possession of an offensive weapon on 2 counts, driving with no tax, MOT or Insurance, being drunk in charge of a vehicle and driving otherwise in accordance of a license. He was sentenced to 4 months in prison and served 2 on the release condition that he was escorted to the airport by his sister who is a lecturer at the university of Cambridge, sent home and not to return to the United Kingdom. He then let the country

He came back to Clacton in an attempt to track us down again and was seen outside my aunt's house. Essex Police had intelligence that he had returned and had informed all officers deployed from Tendring and Colchester Borough Districts. He was then arrested again and released on bail.

This was the point he had made the decision that it was no use fighting anymore and left the country. 1 week later at around 10:30 pm my niece was born and on the following day, my grandfather perished.

On the day my grandfather died, my mum had received a call from my grandmother in the afternoon to inform her that he had collapsed, and they needed help to get him up. He was moved onto the carpet to prevent him from getting too cold. They had called paramedics and my mum was carrying out Cardiopulmonary Resuscitation (CPR) on him. By about 18:30 pm, he was pronounced dead. This had affected the entire family. Personally, I saw him as my father figure because he was an inspiration.

My father never returned to England and my mum had an injunction order to prevent him from entering the Tendring District. We had also had an order put in place specifying that he was only to see us when accompanied by a social worker and 2 police officers with a minimum arming of tasers and visits were only to take place in Colchester or further afield to keep the injunction in order. This information was passed on to the school which I had attended, and the school attended by my brother. In our paperwork at school, there was a note of this which also said, he was not to see us and to call the police upon sight of him.

My brother had developed epilepsy from the trauma of the events that had happened up to this point. One day we were informed that my father was seen in the local area. My brother instantly rushed to the window to vomit. As this has happened, he has hit his shoulder on the window frame and dislocated his shoulder which was followed by an epileptic seizure. At the time, I was scared but was not affected in any such way that my brother was.

I had never seen my brother have a seizure and one day he had laid on the floor and I was worried. He had then begun convulsing and had 3 seizures. I was scared. I was 11 at the time and was crying to the paramedics on the phone. The paramedic on the phone wouldn't let me go until the ambulance had arrived to make sure I didn't go into shock.

CHAPTER 2: BULLYING

The bullying had started during the divorce of my parents. The bullying was predominantly aimed at me being mixed race because at that point, there was 1 other mixed-race family in the area and they were my cousins. I had been called a nigger, a coon, told to go back to my own country and various other racial slurs. These had affected me horrendously. I would never want to go back to school.

One particular day, still during the divorce, I was told "you are a nigger and your dad is a dirty black cunt". Due to this and the circumstances surrounding the situation, I had lost my temper and broke the perpetrators nose and was almost expelled from school.

My mum had been called into the school for a meeting and she had explained to them that she had told me to hit them because the issue was repeatedly being reported to the school, who had taken no action to prevent it.

I was then removed from the classroom and was sent to help the teachers look after the younger students because they had deemed that to be the most suitable solution to the issue at hand. The bullying had stopped at this point, so I thought.

As I progressed into my first year of secondary school, thee bullying had continued and again, was for me being mixed race. It had been reported to the school who had taken no action. There were constant attempts made to stop the bullying. None of these worked, and it had continued and got worse every day.

I then proceeded into my third year of secondary school and the bullying was still going on and had made me feel terrible about going to school and at points it even made me question is it worth living if I'm hated to this extent just for being mixed race. Although at this point, I never told anyone and just kept it to myself.

I had now had enough of being bullied after a consistent 4 and a half years of it. I had flipped and caused at least £1,500 of damage to the school property while I was fighting the bullies which, was all dealt with very quickly. I had almost been arrested by the school police officer until such time as I threatened the school with an Ofsted report because they had been told about the issues and didn't take any action to stop it. At that point they had insisted it wasn't necessary.

The incidents had all found their way around the school. It was at this point that all the bullying had instantly stopped and some of the bullies wanted to be friends with me. I was civil with them but, after everything they had put me through, there was no way I was able to be friends with them.

Bullying does not happen only in schools. People can be bullied in the workplace or even at home. The person who is bullying the other may not necessarily see it as they are being a bully, they may think they are joking with the person and are unaware of how it's truly making the person feel. Another reason people may bully others is that they were once bullied themselves and are trying to fit in or to show that they can have dominance over others. They plan on proving this to others so much that they lose sight of how it made them feel and that they are now making another person feel exactly the same as they once did. They become so concentrated on proving to themselves that they can overcome the bullying and they can also be dominant that they lose sight of where they've been in their journey to where they currently are.

CHAPTER 3: SEXUAL ASSAULT

Just before I had seen red while being bullied, we had taken in a foster child. This was my cousin who had been removed from his own home. One day I was helping him to tidy some things in his room and the door had to be closed due to a built-in cupboard which was right behind the door.

While I was helping him to tidy his room, I had my back turned to him because we were in different parts of the room. I've then felt someone push me and turned as I fell on to the bed and saw it was him. I was then sexually assaulted by him. This had happened on 3 separate occasions with different circumstances each time.

The last time, we went downstairs for dinner and my mum asked if I was ok and I've said that I was because I was scared of so many things that could have happened. I then went straight upstairs to bed. She followed me upstairs because I was acting differently to normal. She asked me again and I said that I was ok again. She then came in and closed the door and said to me "I know there is something wrong because you're not yourself" and I said no I'm ok as my eyes started to fill with tears. She replied to me "What happened in his room, did he do something to you?".

I just burst into tears and couldn't talk, and she said: "right, I'm gonna have him taken away". The next day I returned from school to find boxes around the house and I asked my mum what was going on. She replied, "he's been taken away". We then found out that social services had assigned me a social worker and informed the police who had assigned a detective to us. The social worker and police both turned up to speak to me, my mum and my aunt. They both spoke to them and I refused to talk. I wanted to but couldn't.

It was then that Thurrock Borough Council social services had told us that they knew about him doing it before coming to us. In fact, he had 3 previous victims to me. They hadn't told my mum until the incident happened and my mum was devastated.

I've lived every day since the day it happened feeling like what happened was my fault like I should have stopped him or done something. I've also felt dirty for it and have had to use water in baths that are excessively hot to the extent I can't feel anything when I get out of it and my skin is bright red. I have also had severe trust issues since this day, particularly with males. I have only recently stopped waking up in the middle of the night with night terrors because of it and have also recently managed to start sleeping with my lights off. I was having to be taken out of school for police interviews to support the investigation.

Even now, I feel the same way and am repeatedly told that it was not my fault. I have however, recently been able to stop using water in baths that is too hot. I did not ask for the incident to happen and did not instigate it in any way. People who have suffered sexual assault need to know that they are not alone and that they have no need to be ashamed of what happened to them. It is the attacker that should be ashamed because they have completely changed someone's life with no consideration of the victim's thoughts or their feelings.

Sexual assault is any unwanted act of touching a person's genitals. Sexual assault is not consented and is more common than one would expect. Sexual assault can be committed by any person and can happen to any person. In 2017 145,397 sexual offences were committed in England and wales. That figure reflects approximately 17 sexual offences every hour. The statistics for females are higher but it is unclear as to whether the reasoning is because less men report it, or men are less vulnerable.

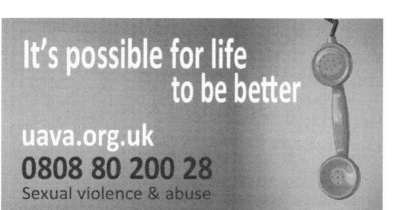

It's possible for life
to be better

uava.org.uk
0808 80 200 28
Sexual violence & abuse

CHAPTER 4: MEDICAL PROBLEMS

Shortly after the assault, I started having seizures. It is still unclear as to whether the 2 are linked. I was initially accused of attention seeking by the doctor at Colchester General Hospital. I was then diagnosed with epilepsy by a paediatric neurologist for which, I was then started on a course of Sodium Valproate (Epilim) which, had made the seizures worse. The dosage was then increased from 500 mg per day, gradually to 2000 mg per day. This had changed the seizures I had.

When I first started having seizures, I would become unconscious and then be disoriented when I was awake again. However, due to the course of incorrect medication, they had then progressed. I would become unconscious and wake up but still be in the seizure at which time, I would get up and start breaking things and attacking those who grabbed me to try to help me. I was having to be restrained by the police before I could be taken to the hospital at the age of 14 and would end up with cut wrists from the handcuffs and head injuries from keep headbutting the concrete floor.

After these incidents, I was taken to a mental health centre under voluntary section during which time, I was examined by mental health nurses and therapists, who had stated that I did not have psychosis. Upon returning to Colchester Hospital, I was given a diagnosis of NMDA encephalitis Receptor B (Anti NMDA receptors) and was asked to submit another blood test for confirmation and was asked by the neurologist if I would have a lumbar puncture. The confirmation test had returned as positive which had then eliminated the need to have a lumbar puncture.

Anti NMDA Receptors are linked with tumours and swelling of the brain and is a life-threatening condition. In the event the patient becomes ill with anything as simple as the common cold, they may be susceptible to their brain swelling, causing them to either be in a coma, intensive care or can possibly cause death. It is still unclear if this condition is hereditary but, the condition is very rare. In the UK, there are a very few people known to have this condition. At the current time, as far as I know, regional hospitals cannot test for this and the blood samples are, therefore required to be sent to Cambridge to be tested.

Many symptoms accompany the Anti-NMDA receptors. One of these is behavioural outbursts and irritability. This may cause the person to suddenly change from happy to angry or sad or any other normal emotion however to an unreasonable level. In addition to this, one of the other effects is sleep dysfunction which, can take it's forming in either excessive sleeping, not sleeping enough or constantly being tired or fatigued. Another ramification of this diagnosis is to be excessively hyperactive. This would give people an irrational amount of energy, strength or the ability to do things they may otherwise not be able to do. Hypersexuality may also occur. This may cause the patient's sex drive to rapidly increase sometimes by a large amount and other times by only a little.

Additional issues which accompany Anti-NMDA receptors are changes in behaviour, deterioration of the patient's cognitive capacity or ability and abnormal speech may develop. Other common hindrances are confusion and short-term memory deficits. These have currently been present in around 95% of the patients of this condition.

I was put through multiple CT scans, an EEG, a sleep-deprived EEG, an MRI, ultrasound scans, x-rays and a video telemetry test in order to investigate the cause of the problems I was facing.

During a Computed Tomography (CT) scan, the patient will be placed on a sliding plate which, will insert them into a tunnel-looking device. Once the radiographer is satisfied with the positioning, they will then activate the machine. This will use x-rays to construct a 3-dimensional image of the interior of the body. The procedure is painless and takes up to 30 minutes.

An Electroencephalogram (EEG) is a test which consists of the patient sitting in a chair and will have electrodes attached to their head using a putty type of glue which washes out. There are many types of EEG test. This is the standard test which is used to investigate memory problems and seizures. The sleep-deprived EEG has the same premise with the exception being that you must not sleep for a minimum of 24 hours prior to the test and the brain-waves will then be monitored.

A Magnetic Resonance Imaging test (MRI) has a very similar premise to the CT scan however, the MRI uses a powerful magnetic field, allowing it to produce a more detailed image of soft body tissue. Unlike the CT scan, MRI does not use any form of x-ray or any other type of radiation. Within an MRI, the patient cannot be in possession of any metallic items due to the strength of the magnetic field.

An ultrasound test is most commonly used to inspect the growth and progression of a foetus within a pregnant woman's womb. However, they are also used to test for tumours. The ultrasound can detect tumours that are both malignant and benign. The ultrasound is a generic scan which can be used for a wide variety of medical investigations.

X-rays can be taken of any part of the body. They will use either alpha or beta rays. The type used will depend on the type of tissue required to be inspected. Beta rays are stronger than alpha rays and an excessive amount of exposure can lead to radiation sickness, however, this is very rare because the radiographers are trained to a high level to ensure the prevention of this.

A Video Telemetry test consists of the patient undergoing an EEG through the course of 48-96 hours. During this time, they will also be video recorded in the main bedroom within the hospital. The camera will not be in the bathroom and the patient cannot shower during this time because the putty will dissolve, rendering the test incomplete and therefore, inadequate for usage during the remainder of the investigation.

These tests can be used for a variety of different diagnosis but most of them are well known for one particular diagnosis or testing for a specific reason.

The seizures were diagnosed as non-epileptic seizures following visits by specialist neurologists due to the case being so rare and unique. There is no medication and no cure for this diagnosis. This is because the initial discovery of the Anti-NMDA Receptors was in 2007.

I was then suffering from symptoms identical to those of a depressed bipolar with issues conversing and meeting new people. I had visited my GP surgery's nurse and was told: "you have to take control of your mental health before you get yourself sectioned or arrested". I then self-referred to Mind who had given me an assessment and diagnosed me with depression, social anxiety, post-traumatic stress disorder (PTSD) and disruptive mood dysregulation disorder (DMDD).

Depression is possibly the most common mental health problem and for that reason, may not be taken as seriously as it should be. When I had visited my GP, I was prescribed with Sertraline. I had taken them for 2 weeks, complying with the regular dose. However, they seemed to be making me a lot more aggressive. I then stopped taking them and informed the doctor and they were not willing to help any more than prescribe me more anti-depressants.

Social anxiety is another very common mental health problem which is treated as more trivial than it should be. Social anxiety can cause hyperventilation, and if the patient suffers from asthma, they may be caused to have an asthma attack. Otherwise, they may have panic attacks. I suffered very badly with the panic attacks and found myself not breathing and almost becoming unconscious due to lack of Oxygen whilst the panic attack was occurring.

The post-traumatic stress disorder (PTSD) has caused me to have night terrors amongst other issues. This originated from the sexual attack I encountered at 13 years old. Psychiatrists find it very difficult to diagnose PTSD. this is because they must rely solely on their observations of the patient alongside what the patient tells them. Another issue which, accompanies PTSD of this origin is that I have found it very difficult to sleep at night with the light switched off. I have also experienced severe trust issues with males, in particular, following the attack because one would assume, they can trust any of their family to keep them safe and not let anyone harm them.

DMDD carries with it many different issues. One of which is cognition problems. People who have DMDD find it difficult to carry out some tasks which many others may not. An additional defect is the temperament of the patient. I have found myself becoming irrationally angry or upset over a trivial matter. On some occasions, it may occur without any stimulus and causes the patient to say and do things which, they later regret. An example is that previously I have had no provocation and have become irrationally angry and have headbutted a brick wall, causing me to have a concussion for 3 weeks. I have also confronted and argued with people, even those who are close to me, sometimes for no reason.

During the Christmas period of 2016 I had become ill and started to vomit every time I was eating food or drinking. I then decided I wasn't going to eat or drink in around January time. I went for 1 month with no food or drink and had woke up in the morning and my tongue had stuck to the top of my mouth, preventing me from breathing. Had I have been asleep for around 10 minutes longer, I would have died from lack of Oxygen. My mum had then said: "today you're either eating or I'm taking you to the hospital and you will be fed there." I agreed to eat a little bit. I had been referred to be investigated for cancer in my digestive system. During this investigation I had a colonoscopy and a prostate exam. These tests were carried out on the lower Gastrointestinal tract (GI).

A colonoscopy is a methodical procedure during which, the patient will be provided strong laxatives 3 days prior to the exam. When they are taken for the lower GI test, they will be sedated and put on Entonox (gas & air or laughing gas). A small camera will then be inserted into the anus and pushed part of the way up the intestines to examine the colon for tumours.

A prostate exam is another lower GI test which, tests for any anomalous lumps on the prostate. A chaperone will be present in this exam. To carry out a prostate exam, the doctor will first pump air into the anus. He will then insert his finger into the patient's anus and feel the prostate for any tumours or any swelling that may occur.

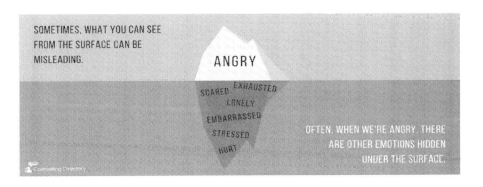

SOMETIMES, WHAT YOU CAN SEE FROM THE SURFACE CAN BE MISLEADING.

ANGRY

SCARED EXHAUSTED
LONELY
EMBARRASSED
STRESSED
HURT

OFTEN, WHEN WE'RE ANGRY, THERE ARE OTHER EMOTIONS HIDDEN UNDER THE SURFACE.

Counselling Directory

CHAPTER 5: UNEMPLOYMENT

I suspect that my medical history had a part to play within my unemployment. I had been unemployed for months, working the doors on Saturday nights. This was my only means of living at the time. At this time, I would have to make £40 feed me every week. However, since then, I have built myself back up by transferring to another company which, gave me Friday and Saturday nights which was earning me £80 per week. From this, I have still encountered many rejections from various companies ranging from working on train tracks to being an apprentice solicitor.

I was visiting the Jobcentre plus weekly for appointments however, they had said that the £80 per week that I was earning was a livable weekly wage and would not pay any money which in my case was fine because I am staying with a relative and have no fixed expenses whereas, others might not be and would need extra money to be able to get by with the expenses they averagely pay such as rent or bills.

I have now found a job which, is paying enough for me to live. This is with a large UK-based security company. However, I have been told by some of my colleagues that I have more potential than security because of my high level of qualifications. The main question is… Am I worth more? And the answer is yes. Anyone who can qualify in something must have the mentality that they are worth the position for which, they are qualified. Speaking from experience, until you appreciate yourself and believe in yourself or you have very good and supportive friends, no one else will.

CHAPTER 6: HOMELESSNESS

During the summer of 2018, I was made homeless. At this current time, I was in a seasonal job as bar staff at one of the local caravan parks. This, however, came to an end when the season ended in November.

Tendring District Council had refused me any support with housing because they said: "with no income, you will not be able to pay the rent every month". I had then visited social services who had said "although you are a vulnerable adult, we cannot help you because you are over 18 and out of education which gives you full adult responsibility for your own wellbeing. Had you have been the primary caregiver to a child under 18, we would be able to house you".

I was made homeless due to my mum having to move in with her partner to attend university because she would not have been able to survive without the secure income during this period. I had asked her to put me on the tenancy of the housing association property we were residing in at the time to allow me to take over the tenancy for the house and she was unable to because of the policy of the housing association. At this point, I was sleeping on a different sofa every night for a while and some nights were spent on the streets when I had nowhere to go until eventually my nan had been called by my aunt, who had only found out because I had asked to stay there. My nan called me and said she was picking me up in the morning and to get all of my things ready. Since then, she has helped me to find a job and is allowing me to live with her in order to improve myself and my prospects of life.

Homelessness currently affects 1 in 200 people in the UK who range across any ages, however, 30% of all homeless people are between the ages of 36 and 45. Although it does not represent a large amount being that 1.06% of all 16-25-year olds are sleeping rough, this equates to 83,000 in the UK alone. These do not include those that are in sheltered accommodation but is only those who will be sleeping in the streets tonight as every other night in the UK. The average waiting time for a council property is around 10 years which, often leaves people homeless for this time. However, the other option is housing benefit in private accommodation which requires the person to have a permanent job with a minimum of 16 hours per week contracted which, cannot be obtained without proof of address and therefore leaving the person with no address to prove in order to get the job.

Social Services had sent me to the council insisting they do not house and are not responsible for vulnerable adults. The council housing had refused me due to a lack of income and sent me to jobcentre plus. However, jobcentre plus said that I was earning a sufficient wage to live and would not supply me with any additional money and suggested I return to Tendring District Council of Essex County Council. This was when I decided I would do it without their help. It was extremely hard and takes a lot of willpower but being stubborn nobody could convince me otherwise.

Street link, the charity for which, I have provided the contact details below will not house people. They are not a housing association and are there to provide advice to those who need it regarding what further steps they need to take in order to be rehomed.

CHAPTER 7: NEGATIVE SOLUTIONS

There are various negative solutions which patients with mental health or others in similar situations to any of those that I have described may use. These will allow the mental health problems to consume your personality and you as a person. They should not be used and have been used by myself at points in which, I felt there was no other way because there was no one willing to help me apart from some of my friends. I had felt enclosed in a black hole which never seemed to brighten up. It was as if I was walking through a tunnel with a torch and the light had gone out. There was no way out, where was the light, the walls, the exit, how do I turn back the way I came? The answer was with my friends, some which I had entered the tunnel with and others that I had met in there. Of course, this is a metaphor and I was never actually stuck in a tunnel.

The first of these negative solutions is suicide. Committing suicide can be done in many forms and is used when people do not feel they have another way out and feel that life is not worth living because of all the things they have going on. The form of suicide I had attempted on multiple occasions was asphyxiation. On one of the occasions, I could feel myself slipping away as my body starved of Oxygen and received a message which lit up my phone and showed a picture of my niece. When I saw her, I couldn't do it to her, she means the world to me and it would destroy her if she could never see me again because my sister has always told me that my niece asks when she can see me because I'm her favourite uncle. Another reason people would attempt suicide is that they may feel unloved. During my time of difficulty, I was feeling this and I have found when someone says it to you, it makes you feel better about yourself which, as odd as it may seem, is why I personally say it to my friends because they say it back and it makes you realise, even though it's as a friend, you are loved. Every person is loved by someone whether it's as a friend, boyfriend, girlfriend, son, daughter, cousin, parent etc. everyone is loved.

The second negative solution I'd like to cover is self -harm. People self-harm for several reasons. One of these is that they may feel something needs to take the impact of the situation and the only thing they have control over is themselves. Others may self-harm because they feel the physical pain can distract them from the emotional pain they are suffering. Self-harm takes a few forms. The most common and most thought of is cutting. There is a common misconception that one direction is for attention and the other is for results. If somebody is self-harming, they are completely lost in their troubles and cannot see the way out of them.

Another form of self-harm is hitting and headbutting walls. I personally, have used this method whilst I was in a severe struggle. I have caused damage to my hands and had countless amounts of concussions from doing this. We do not do this because we think it makes us look tough. We do it because we feel we are worth no more than the pain that is inflicted to ourselves. Some of these damages to my hands are broken fingers and even cuts that have kept bleeding for over 48 hours regardless of all my attempts to stop the bleeding.

Some people turn to drugs and alcohol as their solution to their issues. This is a negative way of attempting to deal with the issues at hand and will never get rid of the problems they are currently facing but, will arise new ones medically and mentally. The prolonged abuse of drugs and alcohol can lead to dependency and may also cause Korsakoff syndrome which is a memory disorder caused by the deficiency of thiamine (Vitamin B1). From the perspective of drugs, the abuse of them can cause an alteration of the gene expressions and the brain circuitry.

Telling people, you're ok when you're not is an additional negative solution to mental health issues. Sometimes just talking about things can make people feel better because whilst it is being conversed about, it then starts to be rationalised in your mind with the assistance of the friend's advice. Sometimes people just need to vent and rather than advice are looking for a person to just listen, so they can put their thoughts and feelings across. If they cannot do this, it may be frustrating for them, causing them to advance to another negative solution.

An additional negative solution I am going to list is allowing the mental health problems consume you and your life. Mental health problems are a part of life and are not rare. 25% of the UK's population will experience mental health problems within the period of a year. Some may take years to overcome and some could take weeks. My personal experience with this is that I would wake up in the morning and not want to go out and so would lock all the doors in the house and close the curtains to make it look like there was no one home. I would also not answer my phone or the house phone and this would go on for days, sometimes weeks at a time. In addition to this, I used to not answer the door. I have had my college send the police to my house on one of these occasions because I was absent for 2 weeks with no contact made and my mum was away on holiday so did not know what was occurring. They had tried sending the school bus to check on me and I did not open the door to them either. I wasn't going to answer the door to the police when they knocked until they shouted through the door "police, open the door or we will force entry to the property". I then checked through the spyglass on the door. When I opened the door, I knew one of the officers but not the other, so I had allowed him into the house, but the other officer was made to stay outside because of how vulnerable I was feeling at the time against anyone I did not know.

Taking an overdose of any type of drug is also a very negative way of dealing with mental health problems which is extremely painful and will make the patient very ill. The main premise of taking an overdose is to commit suicide. Personally, I have thought about taking an overdose of various legal drugs which I know would have killed me. One of my friends begged me not to take the planned overdose because I had planned to also take medication to prevent the excretion of faeces which would have meant I couldn't pass the various medicines and so, they would be stuck in my system until they had the 'desired' effect. I had planned to take this overdose because things were getting too much for me to handle and I felt like nobody cared. When my friend called me and was on the phone to me begging me not to do it, I replied with "nobody cares anyway. My problems are getting too much, I can't deal with them anymore". He has then said: "we all care, all of your friends love you… I love you". I broke down on the phone and said: "I need help". He then took me to the hospital with his mum and they took me to a mental health assessment. I apologized to him and he answered: "it's ok, you're not well. Let's get you some help.". Drugs overdoses are bad and should never be taken. As proven in this section, people do care regardless of the dark thoughts convincing you that they don't.

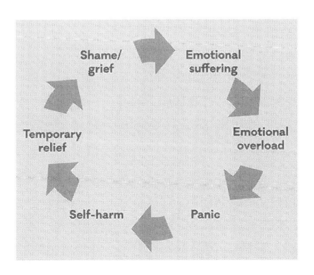

Chapter 8: Positive solutions

Alongside the negative solutions stated, there are also positive solutions which will assist in managing mental health problems. The positive resolutions will allow the patient, not only to manage their mental health but to also attempt to get to the root of their mental health problems in order to try and avoid them becoming worse later, and to eventually allow them to overcome their mental health problems. It is by no means a fast process at all, it will take time.

The first positive solution is to accept that you need it and ask for help. Until the point you accept that you need help, you will always be in denial about having mental health problems. Asking for help is possibly the hardest part about dealing with mental health problems but, until the time as you can ask your friends, family or the mental health services for help, you will not be able to overcome your mental health problems. In my case, having 4 mental health problems, there were people that feared me or tried to avoid me purely because of the way that my mood could change instantly, or I could even wake up in a bad mood sometimes. Whilst asking for help, the patient needs to fully open up to those that are trying to help them. Show them your emotions, tell them how it has affected your life and the relationships you have or had, as the case may be. Make sure they know all the details because it is only when they have the information that they can then start, not to know how you feel but to understand how you feel and what you're going through and experiencing. It is only at this time that they can help you. This is a positive solution not only to mental health, but also to dealing with addiction.

Another positive solution is to have good friends around you who are willing to help you and listen to you. Friends are very accepting and do all they can to help you get through your time of need. Personally, I've had a friend who has sat up with me all night and spoke to me and talked me out of committing suicide because I felt that low that it was the only way out. He knows that I'm very grateful now for what he has done for me and told me "I would never be able to live with myself if something happened and I didn't do anything". At the time, I didn't know I meant that much to my friends, in fact, I thought they just wouldn't notice at all. However, that night changed my perception of it all and I realised that my friends do care and will help me and that I mean more to them than I know. This intends to show that everyone means more to people then then they realise.

Another of the most important solutions for a positive outcome would be to accept the help that is offered. Trust those who are trying to help you, as hard as it may be, it is a barrier that needs to be overcome. People refuse offered help for a number of reasons such as embarrassment or they don't feel they are worth the person's help or trouble. However, they are, everyone is worth the help they are offered and more. Anyone who is offered help should take all the help they can get because it's until then they will not truly be able to solve their mental health problems. Most people will turn down the help the first time they are offered because they don't want to bother the person that has offered but if the person has offered, they already are bothered… about the fact they are seeing their friend, family member or patient being led slowly to the array of mental health problems and may be worried about losing the relationship they have with the patient. This is because when people have mental health problems they change for the worse, they will usually be very needy with their friends and then suddenly not speak to them for a few weeks and then go back to being needy with them. Most friends can't handle how needy people with mental health problems get because they are always conversing in some way until the patient stops for a few weeks and doesn't speak a word to them and no one hears from that person during this time. Some people assume the worst and others assume the patient needs some space but, although at the time the ones who assume the worst seem to be a pain, they are doing their best to look out for you and showing that they do truly care for you and your problems.

CONTACT DETAILS

If you have experienced any of the issues in the book please do not face them alone, there are various agencies who can be contacted to help.

I would like to emphasize women are not the only sufferers of domestic violence and would urge everyone who is subject to domestic violence to seek help. Men are just a vulnerable to domestic violence as women are. The predominant reason for the statistics for men being at lower risk of domestic violence is because less men report it than women do. In addition, females can also be sexual attackers and both males and females can be sexually assaulted by males and by females. The risk is the same for men and women. No gender, age, identity or race is exempt from the possibility of being sexually assaulted.

If you think someone has taken an overdose of drugs of any type, please call 999 straight away. They need help, if they are at the stage that they have lost consciousness following an overdose, they need help straight away. Do not take the advice of some online webpages which say the best thing is to leave them because it's not that they took the choice to overdose. They felt there is nothing left for them and that no one is there for them. Get them the medical and mental help they need and remind them that you care about them, let them know that they matter to you.

In addition, if you feel somebody is a genuine risk to either themselves or anyone else, call 999 ask for police and ambulance and explain to them that the person is a risk to themselves and others and the best path for them is to be taken into professional care under section 4 of the Mental Health Act. This will allow them to take the patient to a care centre or hospital ward in order to assess them for a maximum of 72 hours. If they are proven to be a risk, they will then be conveyed to section 3 which under the mental health act, will mean they are then taken into the custody of healthcare professionals, who specialise in mental health. The best way to carry this out is to attempt to convince the person to attend care under voluntary section prior to calling the emergency services.

Domestic Violence
Victim support:
08081689111

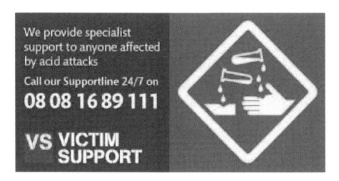

Police
Non-emergency police:
101
In an emergency, always call 999

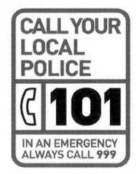

Homelessness
Street Link: 0300 5000 914

Connecting rough sleepers to local services
0300 500 0914 www.streetlink.org.uk

41413352R00031

Printed in Poland
by Amazon Fulfillment
Poland Sp. z o.o., Wrocław